POTTY TRAINING
IN 3 DAYS

The Step-by-Step Plan for a
Clean Break from Dirty Diapers

BRANDI BRUCKS

Foreword by Dr. Fredric Daum

Illustrations by Cleonique Hilsaca

ALTHEA
PRESS

For general information on our other products and services or to obtain technical support, please contact our Customer Care Department within the U.S. at (866) 744-2665, or outside the U.S. at (510) 253-0500.

Althea Press publishes its books in a variety of electronic and print formats. Some content that appears in print may not be available in electronic books, and vice versa.

Illustrations © Cleonique Hilsaca/Illozoo

ISBN: Print 978-1-62315-790-6 | eBook 978-1-62315-791-3

POTTY TRAINING IN 3 DAYS

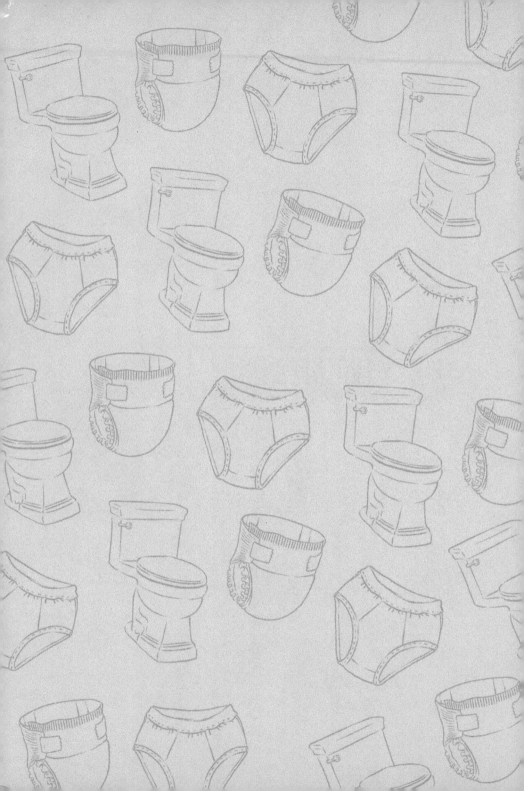

I DEDICATE THIS BOOK
TO MY HUSBAND, WHO NEVER
ONCE TOLD ME MY JOB
WAS WEIRD.

CONTENTS

after the three days

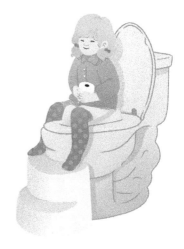

FOREWORD

AS DIRECTOR OF THE Bowel Management Program at a university teaching hospital in New York and medical director of the Encopresis Center, I toilet train more than 1,000 children each year. These are children ages 3 to 12 who have functional constipation (stool withholding, fecal soiling, encopresis) and urinary tract issues. All the children I work with have one thing in common: They are behaviorally resistant to toilet training.

In my experience, following a well-conceived and well-structured plan is the key to toilet-training success. With successful toilet training, your child will have a better self-image and better focus. When you can throw the diapers away after just three days, the result is a beaming, happy, confident child.

In this book, Brandi Brucks has defined the essence of potty training. She understands that the parents' mind-set is what makes or breaks toilet training. Brandi reminds me of the best teachers I had in school who emphasized consistency, firmness, and structure. They were the bosses. Brandi's challenge to doctors who advise that you "wait until your child is ready" is unique and refreshing. She encourages parents to take command and enables them to make good decisions. You don't need to ask your child for permission. You can get it done!

This book is a must for every parent's bookshelf. It reminds parents how rewarding potty training can be. Follow Brandi's suggestions. Look at the summaries she provides. They are a wonderful guide. Like Brandi says, take charge, be optimistic, and always be encouraging. When it comes to toilet training, don't be a friend. Be a parent.

Dr. Fredric Daum
Mineola, New York

INTRODUCTION

Knock, knock.

The door opens slowly and a woman in her sixties gives me a confused look.

"Can I help you?" she asks.

"Yes, I'm Brandi, your potty-training consultant. May I come in?"

"You don't look old enough. I was expecting someone a grandmother's age."

"Well, I am definitely not a grandmother, but I can assure you I have a lot of experience. I have a master's degree in education, and I have worked with children for many years."

"I didn't know you could go to school to learn how to potty train."

"You can't. I just accidentally became really good at it."

AND THAT IS A TRUE STORY. I had always dreamed of becoming a teacher, which is why I earned my MA in elementary education from Simmons College in Boston, Massachusetts. Immediately after graduation, I moved to Austin, Texas, where I thought I would find my dream job as a teacher. But, shortly after I moved there, there was a statewide hiring freeze for teachers.

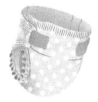

What was I going to do? I started nannying.

Families have changed so much. Years ago, when there were more stay-at-home moms, potty training tended to happen in private, without much discussion. Today, there are more children who grow up with both parents working outside the home. And potty training isn't something every parent has the time (or the desire) to do. Everywhere I went as a nanny, it seemed as if someone needed to be potty trained.

That was my cue.

Never in a million years did I imagine I would potty train other people's children for a living. My clients open their homes to me, and I love spending a few days with different families. It has been such a wonderful experience. I tear up every time one of "my kids" pees on the potty for the first time—although I will deny it!

My biggest joy in writing this book is knowing I can help so many people who feel overwhelmed—or just clueless—about how to potty train their children. You absolutely can teach your child the fundamentals of potty training in three days. In this book, I will give you the confidence to tackle any crappy situation. :-)

Stay strong! You are the parent. You can do this.

before the three days

1 timing is everything

2 always be reasonable

3 learn to speak potty

4 introduce the toilet

5 prepare for the three days

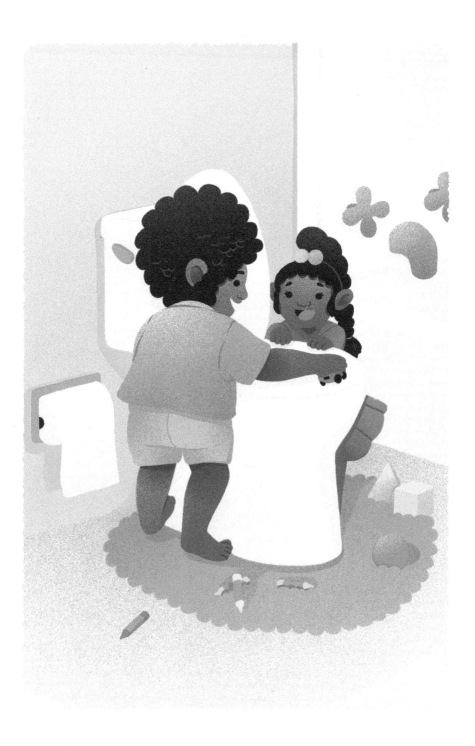

timing is everything

My son seems interested in the bathroom, but he doesn't do anything when I put him on the potty.

My daughter throws a screaming fit when I try to sit her on the toilet.

I put my daughter in underwear, and she peed all over the house— never once in the toilet. What am I doing wrong?

I tried potty training my kid three times, and nothing has worked!

What if I mess this up?

IF THIS IS YOU, TAKE A DEEP BREATH. Relax. I am about to make this whole potty-training thing so easy, you're going to wonder where I have been your whole life. Well, maybe not your whole life, but at least the recent part involving diapers, poop, and pee.

when to start

So you have a kid in diapers and you no longer want the kid to be in diapers. Great!

You both are ready to venture into the crazy world of Toddler-dom, which means your baby is no longer a baby.

But Little Bob will always be my baby!

Yes, I know, but as far as potty training is concerned, Little Bob needs to be a "big boy" now.

Every child is different, of course, so while there are quite a few signs indicating whether or not your child is ready for potty training, making sure she is *developmentally* ready is most important. In my experience, if your child is more than two and a half years old, there is a good chance she is ready for potty training. If she is three years old, she is *definitely* ready. At that age, children have better control over their bladders and bodies and can cognitively understand the process.

The youngest child I have potty trained was 21 months old; the oldest was four and a half years old. The 21-month-old had only one accident during her potty-training time, and she was so young, she will never remember a time in her life when she was in diapers. The four-and-a-half-year-old, on the other hand, spent all his toddler years in diapers and pull-ups, which made the potty-training process much more difficult and emotional. I had to spend a good portion of our time together making him feel comfortable about wearing underwear, instead of focusing on actually peeing on the potty. While you may not be ready to take the potty-training plunge with your two-year-old (which is okay), it will get harder with each passing month.

five signs your kid is ready

Consider these signs as you ponder your child's potty-training potential:

1. SHE KNOWS WHEN IT'S TIME TO BE CHANGED.

If your child is coming to you wanting to be changed after she has gone to the bathroom in her pull-up or diaper, then your child is ready to be potty trained *right now*. This is her way of telling you, "Hey, I don't like this feeling." Actually, if this is your child, you are pretty lucky because she will probably pick up on potty training very quickly. She wants to feel comfortable. And she already understands the first concept of potty training: Being wet or dirty in our pants is a yucky feeling!

2. SHE CAN HOLD HER BLADDER.

When your child is trained, you will expect her to keep her underwear dry for at least an hour at a time. If she is still peeing frequently, this could mean she isn't quite ready developmentally. If your child has some wetness in her diaper every 30 minutes or sooner, this usually means her urinary tract system has not developed enough to "hold it" when she needs to pee.

However, if your child shows other signs of being ready, perhaps she is simply peeing so much because she's drinking too many fluids. Try giving her less to drink.

3. SHE DOESN'T HAVE HARD POOP.

Your child's bowel movements are a big sign as to whether or not she is ready for potty training. Children who tend to have hard poop often become constipated, which can cause pain when they go to the bathroom. Even one painful bowel movement can cause irrational bathroom fear in your child. That fear may seem irrational to us, since we know everyone poops on the potty and it's going to be okay, but our children don't know that. Even if they have successfully pooped on the potty once before, they are still not 100 percent sure they will be okay.

If your child is constipated or has painful BMs, it is important for her see a pediatrician. Many children are put on medication, such as MiraLAX, by their pediatrician to help pass bowel movements. If you take this path with your child, make sure she is not having hard stools for at least two weeks before you start the potty-training process.

4. SHE CAN FOLLOW DIRECTIONS.

Although it's not the most important sign of readiness, following simple directions is a sign parents often do not think about. Potty training is a sequence of steps your child has to follow to succeed. If she can understand one or two directions, then she should be able to understand your potty-training directions: Walk to the bathroom. Pull down your pants. Step on the stool. Sit on the potty, and so on.

5. SHE SHOWS INTEREST.

And, of course, showing interest or asking questions about the bathroom is a big sign of readiness. This means your child is starting to notice things that happen in this room aside from just taking a bath! Common signs include watching when you use the toilet, wanting to flush, wanting to look inside the toilet, and so on. Children don't always know how to ask the right questions, so even having your kiddo drop some toys into the toilet is a sign she is ready to learn more. Don't you love fishing crayons and cars out of the toilet?

IS YOUR KID READY?

In general, your child is ready for potty training when at least three of the following five things are true:

1. Your child tells you she needs to be and/or wants to be changed when she is wet or dirty.
2. She can remain dry for up to two hours at a time.
3. She has one or two bowel movements during the day, and they're not very hard.
4. She is able to follow simple directions.
5. She shows interest in the bathroom.

if you start early

While the golden age for potty training seems to be between two and a half and three years old, some children may be ready earlier. My husband's grandmother swears up and down she had all five of her children potty trained before they were even 18 months old, so you can imagine how crazy she thinks my job is! The truth is you can potty train your child at any age—it's just a matter of how much effort you want to put into it.

Training your baby before the age of two is called "elimination communication" or "baby potty training." This is not what I am going to teach you. But just so you know, with this method you try to learn your baby's body cues and hold her over the toilet when she needs to go. This is the way some cultures, such as the Digo tribe in Kenya and Tanzania, potty train their children.

if you start late

If you are potty training your child and she is over the age of three and a half, the process may be a little more difficult for you. Your child may understand your directions and be more physically developed, but you might have to deal with a behavioral aspect of potty training that usually doesn't come into play when you train a child at a younger age.

The less time your child has been in diapers, the easier it will be to transition her to underwear. And, in my experience, children who potty train at an older age need more time to feel comfortable going poop on the potty.

Sometimes older children become emotionally attached to their diapers because it is the only way they have ever felt comfortable going to the bathroom. With older children, you have to be extra confident because three-year-olds (or Threenagers, as they are called these days) tend to throw tantrums to get their way. I have seen a three-year-old throw such a momentous fit that her parents gave up on potty training—even though she was clearly ready for it. Round 1: Kid 1, Parents 0. You have to go into this process knowing you will stick to your guns: *No more diapers!*

if your child is delayed

As I said earlier, making sure your child is developmentally ready for potty training is the most important thing. If your child was born prematurely, has physical or mental challenges, is speech delayed, or has any other developmental challenges, you may need to potty train her later than two and a half. Any developmental delays, even just speech, mean a child's central nervous system is delayed as well. The nervous system overlaps with body parts that are important for potty training, such as the bladder, pelvic floor, and bowels.

always be reasonable

POTTY TRAINING ISN'T AS SCARY as we build it up to be, and, honestly, the more you stress about it, the more your child will pick up on that stress and relate it to the bathroom. This whole process should be as fun as possible—so start telling yourself this *will* be fun, and you *will* be successful!

don't pick a fight

I am going to be brutally honest right now: When I do the potty training for other people, their children do not fight with me at all. The only time a child starts to pick fights or resist potty training is when the parents are home, which tells me a great deal about the discipline in that household. Obviously children behave better for other people than they do for their own parents, because every child knows how to play their parents like a fiddle. You may be thinking, *No way. Little Bob couldn't possibly know how to manipulate me.* Well, he does.

I have witnessed so many mini master manipulators, in fact, that when I come into a client's home to do the potty training, I make it

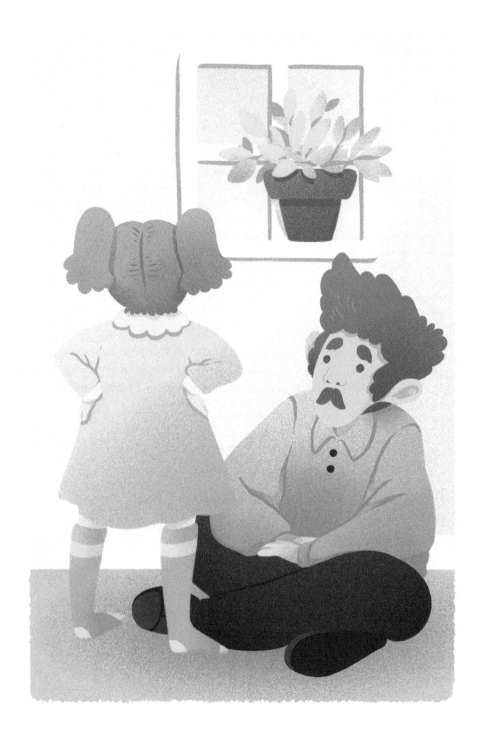

a requirement that the parents leave the home for a bit on Day 1 of training. I spend time with the family beforehand so I can see how a child behaves for her parents, and then I compare that behavior to how she acts when she's alone with me. If I can correct negative behaviors during my alone time with the child, then I know who actually runs the household . . . and most of the time it is the child!

If your child runs your household, she most likely will take control of potty training—when you should control it. Give your child the rules and guidelines, *and stick to them*. Oftentimes, children try to test the limits during new situations. To avoid fighting, be firm with your initial rules.

That said, potty training should be fun! I always encourage my clients to remember this is a big milestone for their children, and they get to be the ones to teach them this important life lesson. Going from diapers to underwear means your baby is no longer a baby—and this should be celebrated. If you get excited, your child will get excited, too.

potty-training myths

There are so many potty-training myths out there. I want to clear those up before I talk about my process. I actually start all my workshops with a little true/false quiz that helps me see where everyone is mentally and lets me know which areas I need to be specific about when discussing my process. Here are some of the most common myths:

1. PLACING A LITTLE POTTY IN VARIOUS PLACES AROUND THE HOUSE ENCOURAGES POTTY TRAINING.

   While I am not sure this a common myth, for some reason, people think this is a perfectly normal thing to do. It is first on my list because this is, honestly, the most common *mistake* I see in my clients' homes. I always have my clients show me around their home before we start training, and I have seen little toilets in the following places: the kitchen, the bathroom, next to the couch in the living room, next to a child's bed, the hallway, and the playroom.

So let me ask you: Do you feel comfortable going to the bathroom in your kitchen? How about in the hallway? Next to your couch while watching TV? *No?* When little toilets are put in these places, you encourage your child to feel comfortable going to the bathroom in other areas of the house, when, really, she should feel comfortable going to the bathroom only in the actual *bathroom*.

One habit you want your child to change during the potty-training process is the one where she feels comfortable peeing and pooping all over the house. When a child is in diapers, she is literally allowed to go to the bathroom wherever and whenever she wants—and then, all of a sudden, we ask her not to. Therefore, it gives a child mixed signals when a little toilet is placed anywhere but in the bathroom.

2. BOYS ARE HARDER TO TRAIN THAN GIRLS.

Statistically, I have trained many more boys than girls, but I find that to be a coincidence. I actually think the girls I have trained have been more challenging. There are many other factors that contribute to how easy training your child will be, including birth order, personality type, and your parenting style.

I have found that the first child or an only child tends to be trained at an older age because this is a parent's first go-around. This usually makes potty training more difficult. Younger siblings get to experience seeing an older sibling use the toilet, and, as the saying goes, "monkey see, monkey do." However, if a younger sibling is babied too much by the parents, sometimes that kiddo enjoys being the baby *so much*, she resists the "big kid" movement that needs to be embraced to be successful with potty training.

Why have I trained so many boys? Almost all the boys I have trained fall into the same personality type. Parents often make the mistake of thinking their child just isn't ready for potty training, when really Little Bob just needed a little extra "kick" in his little pants to get started.

3. YOUR CHILD WILL TELL YOU WHEN SHE IS READY FOR POTTY TRAINING.

In some lucky cases, this is true. In many, many cases, this is *not* true. Don't feel badly if your child isn't that child who one day hops on the toilet and pees on the potty without your prompting. Every time I have potty trained a child older than three, her parents have said to me, "I really thought she would have shown some interest by now." As I have said before, the earlier you train, the easier it is for everyone involved. So, if you're waiting for your child to have an opinion on the matter . . . well, then you've already waited too long because now your child does have an opinion on the matter!

4. PULL-UPS HELP YOU WITH TRAINING.

The only difference between pull-ups and diapers is that diapers have pull-tabs while pull-ups have to be stepped into like a pair of underwear. For some reason that subtle difference has parents flocking to the stores to buy pull-ups, thinking, *Wow! Little Bob is magically going to know how to pull his pants down and go to the bathroom now!* In reality, diapers and pull-ups are made of the same material and feel exactly the same while being worn, which means Little Bob is going to pee in them just like he peed in his diapers.

WHAT PERSONALITY TYPE DOES YOUR CHILD HAVE?

I read a great book a while back called *Personality Plus for Parents: Understanding What Makes Your Child Tick* by Florence Littauer. It really opened my eyes and taught me to look at children in a different way—and, the more children I potty trained and the more children I was around, the more I found I really could place every child into one or two of these personality types, which helps me tailor my approach to each individual child.

Strong-willed, opinionated, ambitious, extrovert

If you have a child with this personality type, it is very important to know how to work with her to reduce the amount of head butting that can occur. This child can sometimes be stubborn, bossy, and unwilling to cooperate if someone *tells* her she needs to do something. She wants to do things when she wants, how she wants, and where she wants. She tends to work things out by herself because she believes she is always right.

On the flip side, this can potentially be the easiest personality type to potty train because the child is often independent and can mostly potty train herself. You need to give the appearance that she has some form of control to avoid argument. Offer choices, but make sure they are *your* choices. For instance, ask whether she would like an apple or a banana for her snack, instead of asking what she *wants* for snack. This eliminates the choice of sugary snacks or the disappointment when she can't have her choice. With potty training, you can offer choices like, "Would you like to sit on the potty by yourself, or would you like some help?"

Life of the party, silly, pleasure seeking, extrovert

This child loves having loads of fun. If you want her to cooperate to her fullest potential, make things exciting. Potty training needs to be a grand event to capture her attention and keep it—otherwise, she'll lose interest quickly. This child loves attention and loves people—so involving more people in the toilet-training process will give her a sense of pride! Take a video of her sharing her exciting news and send it to Mom, Dad, Grandma, the nanny . . . anyone who is special to her.

The negative aspect of this personality type is that love of the limelight! It is sometimes hard when that goes away. This child may regress a little once the special attention wears off, so wean her off the rewards a bit slowly to ease the transition.

Thinker, perfectionist, introvert

You know you have a child with this personality by the constant barrage of "Why?" questions. She isn't asking to be irritating, I promise. This personality is often afraid of change, and, because of that, she requires a lot of information before embarking on new tasks.

So, when potty training this child, supply her with information, and lots of it, *before* you start the process. Explain *what* will happen, *why* it will happen, *how* it will happen, *how long* it will be happening (underpants are forever now), *what you expect* of her, what *reward* can be earned, and so on. This personality is very cautious and won't attempt new things until she thinks she can do them perfectly—which is why it is important to load up on the details before starting.

Laid-back, easy-going, people pleaser, introvert

If you're wondering which personality type is the hardest to train, this is it! This personality generally goes through life doing as little as possible, exerting as little energy as possible. She needs to be told what to do or, more often than not, she won't do it—most likely because she doesn't want to be bothered. This child doesn't always like work because she knows it is *work*, yet she is usually good at taking orders because she likes to please people.

To potty train a child with this personality, you need to guide her constantly and, metaphorically, hold her hand throughout the process. Don't wait for this child to be ready for potty training, because you will wait a long time! Because this child rarely shows interest in potty training, parents often mistake this personality type for "not being ready" when, really, she just needs some extra encouragement.

5. TAKING YOUR CHILD TO THE BATHROOM EVERY 30 MINUTES ENCOURAGES HER TO GO.

Doing this is a surefire way to get your child to hate potty training and resist you in every way possible. I, personally, don't have to go to the bathroom every 30 minutes, and your child most likely doesn't either. Forcing her to do so will only cause frustration. Transitions are difficult for toddlers as it is—creating even more transitions for yourself and your child will hinder your progress.

During the potty-training process, it is important for your child to know what it feels like to have a full bladder. This teaches her how to "hold it." If your child pees every 30 minutes, then you are training her to "need" to go to the bathroom every 30 minutes, instead of holding it and going to the bathroom every couple of hours.

Also, you want to build trust with your child. You want to encourage her to tell you before she needs to go. If you make your child go every 30 minutes, then there is no reason for her ever to communicate with you about it because you will make her sit even if she isn't ready; hence, the frustration emanating from your child.

stick to the plan

Whenever I give potty-training workshops, I tell parents that the absolute first step in potty training is figuring out your plan. Not only should you figure out a solid approach, but everyone in the household should be in on the plan as well. Nothing is more confusing to a toddler than inconsistency. If the parents and the nanny have different bathroom procedures, it can potentially take longer to potty train that child because she must learn two sets of steps, instead of being able to practice one solid, consistent procedure every time.

With my plan, I recommend you set aside two or three whole days for potty training, not a few hours here and a few hours there. I (seriously) had clients who dedicated an entire summer vacation to potty training their son—and who were completely shocked when I ended up training him in about 18 waking hours. This should not be you! Do you fantasize that Little Bob could be out of his diapers by the end of the weekend? Well, your dreams can come true!

While every child is different and learns at a different pace, my plan teaches good bathroom procedures and reinforces positive behavior. After reading this book, you will feel confident and ready to tackle potty training—and have a good idea of the little tricks your kiddo might try to pull on you during this time!

And if your child isn't one of those kids who pick up potty training in 18 hours, that's totally okay! You have to remember you are trying to break your child of one habit (that she has known for years) and teach her a new one. I always tell my clients to stick to the plan for a solid 10 days before stopping or trying something new. Breaking an old habit isn't always easy for every child. Or for anyone.

you are the grown-up

You are the boss, not your child. This may seem like a silly thing to tell you, but how many times have you found yourself arguing or trying to rationalize with your irrational mini-human? Probably more than you would like to admit. (I am in this category, too!)

When my mother was frustratingly trying to potty train me, my father would often have to remind her, *"She is not your boss."* In "Brandi Fashion," I always wanted everything to be my way; however, toddlers do not know what is best for them when it comes to potty training. Not only that, but this is something completely new to them, so, really, their opinion about it should be your opinion about it. This is why you need to be firm and consistent.

Keep calm and carry on! Kids feed off our energy. That's why when Mama ain't happy, ain't nobody happy! Kids will pick up on your frustration, and, if you are showing it about potty training, your kiddo will subconsciously link your negative feelings with going to the bathroom. This creates an irrational fear that will only escalate as the child gets older.

If you are frustrated, take a deep breath. Most times I see parents get frustrated when their child has an accident, but accidents are actually necessary learning opportunities for your child! Your child *is* going to have accidents. Tell yourself this a few times before you even start training; it helps mentally prepare you. So try to keep calm, because this messy time you're about to go through is only a short, temporary phase.

enjoy it

Keep in mind this is bonding time for you and your child. In our busy world, we don't always get one-on-one time with our kids for two or three whole days. You get to help your child reach an important milestone, and, since you'll get to spend so much time with Little Bob, you will have lots of opportunities to snap cute pictures of him in his underpants to use as blackmail for those high school days.

don't give up

Again, do not stop the training before completing 10 full days of this plan. Meaning, from the moment you put your child in underwear on Day 1, follow through with this plan until you have gone through 10 full days. In 3 days you can completely teach your child to pee on the potty with minimal accidents toward the end. It takes longer than 3 days to create a new habit, however. So, wait 10 days until reevaluating your plan if you feel it hasn't worked.

ALWAYS REMEMBER:

» You are the boss!
» As the saying goes . . . keep calm and carry on!
» This is great bonding time for you and your child.
» Don't waver from the plan for at least 10 days.
» You can do this.

A mom came up to me after one of my potty-training boot camp classes and told me how she had tried everything to get her daughter trained, that nothing had worked, and "When I put her in panties, she peed all over the house. It was a disaster." She was traumatized, so she put her child back into diapers. The *mom* was traumatized, not the little girl.

My first question to her was, "Well, how long was she in underpants?"

Her answer? "Forty-five minutes."

I had a good laugh (in my head) when she told me that. Folks, it takes longer than 45 minutes to break a habit! We fall before we walk, and we pee on the floor before we can pee in the toilet. If you are potty training your child who is three right now, remember she has had three years of knowing she is supposed to pee in her diaper, and only a few days of knowing she is now supposed to pee somewhere else—somewhere more inconvenient compared to the portable toilet she has been wearing.

If the plan really isn't working after 10 days, there is usually a specific reason. Most likely it is a behavioral issue, the child isn't developmentally ready, or, I'm sorry to say, you are doing something wrong. Hopefully, by the end of this book, you will know all the things not to do!

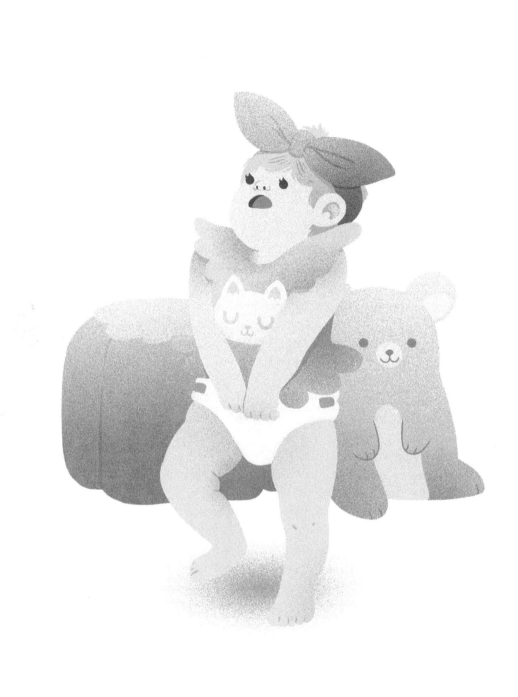

learn to speak potty

HONESTLY, DO YOU REALLY KNOW how your bladder works? Because I definitely didn't until a few years into potty training when I thought, *Duh, of all people, maybe I should know this!*

how does a bladder work?

Your bladder is part of your urinary tract, which also includes your ureters, kidneys, and urethra. The bladder is an organ you can pretty much compare to a balloon that fills up with pee instead of air, and, aside from that, it doesn't do much else. Your kidneys produce your pee, and the way that happens, very simply put, is by your kidneys filtering your blood, which then mixes with water and other waste to create urine. Your urine then travels down two tubelike muscles called ureters. Your ureters have muscles in their walls that are constantly tightening and relaxing, which causes the urine to travel away from the kidneys. If your urine stands still for too long and doesn't travel down your ureters, then you are at risk for developing a kidney infection, which I have had, and I don't wish on anyone!

The other really important body parts that play a role in going to the bathroom are your urethra, the internal and external sphincters, and your pelvic floor. Your urine leaves your bladder and travels through your urethra, where the urine then comes out of your body. Your sphincters are actually more important than you think, as they are the muscles that tighten around your urethra, sort of like a rubber band, to keep your bladder from leaking and having accidents.

Is *pelvic floor* a new term for you? Don't worry. I polled my friends, and no one knew what it was! (My husband thought it was a bone, hehe.) It includes the word *floor* in it for a reason. It provides support for your uterus, bowels, and bladder to lie on, among other things. It is a muscle—so it can be weakened and strengthened. If it becomes too weak, it has to work extra hard to keep the bladder sphincter closed, which means leakage will probably occur. You need to relax this muscle to allow for urination, and most kids just don't realize they can control this until you draw attention to it during potty training.

body language

Kids communicate their wants and needs in many different ways—by talking, pointing, crying, hitting, and so on. You probably know more about your child's moods and desires by her body language than you even realize. Part of potty training is learning, or recognizing, your child's body cues.

Through the years I have found that parents often think their child isn't ready for training because he hasn't come right out and said, "I want to pee on the potty." Little Bob actually doesn't have to be able to talk much to be trained, although it is helpful. When I potty trained my first 21-month-old, she was a bit delayed with her speech, but she was still able to communicate with gestures. Halfway

HOW CHILDREN COMMUNICATE THEIR BATHROOM NEEDS

If you see any of these signs from your child during the potty-training process, it's time to start giving her all those bathroom reminders.

» A panicked expression on her face
» Fidgeting
» Getting angry at you
» Grabbing herself
» Hiding from you when you aren't looking (or even when you are)
» Looking down at her diaper/underwear
» Random crying or fussiness
» Squatting
» Stopping all movement

through training, she walked over to me and patted the front of her diaper, indicating she had to go. This became her sign that she needed to go until her vocabulary was more developed.

Many kids in diapers have a certain spot in the house they have deemed poop-worthy. It is usually a private spot or somewhere she feels really comfortable, such as her bedroom, a closet, behind the couch, in a private corner of the house, or the playroom. If your child does this, make sure she never has the opportunity to be alone in those spots when she needs to go to the bathroom; until she is comfortable consistently using the toilet, she will prefer to poop in her old familiar spots instead.

call it out

There are many things you can talk with your child about, even before you start potty training. If you mentally prepare Little Bob with lots of information, he will have fewer questions and concerns when you start the actual training. Don't start Day 1 of training with everything being new information for him; it will be very overwhelming.

A few weeks before training, it is important to begin drawing your child's attention to her dirty diapers. Many toddlers do not understand the difference between being wet and dry, and knowing this before they start potty training is actually really helpful. Not only that, but you can start putting it into her head that a dirty diaper feels yucky and a clean one feels much better. Every time you change her is a great opportunity for a conversation.

Aside from the new conversations you will have during diaper changing, it's also a really great step to start changing your child while he is standing up, when possible. Potty training is that milestone that evolves your child from a baby to a toddler. When you change a baby, you have to lay him down, but Little Bob isn't a baby anymore. When you change a child standing up, it is more like the process he goes through during training, when he will need to pull his underpants up and down.

WHAT TO SAY

66 Your diaper is wet. Let's get you into a nice, clean diaper. 99

66 Your diaper is dirty. Let's put on a clean one. 99

66 It feels nice to be clean. 99

66 You feel wet. Now you're dry. 99

Allowing your child to accompany you to the restroom is another really good learning experience for her before she starts training. You can explain all you want, but adding the visual aspect certainly makes things clearer. This is also a great way for your child to learn that everyone pees on the potty and it isn't something to be scared of. During this time, you can explain what is going on so she understands.

WHAT TO SAY

66 Mommy drank a lot of water, and now my body is telling me I need to go potty. Let's go together. 99

66 Do you hear that sound? Mommy put all her pee in the potty. 99

66 Help me flush my pee down the toilet. Say, 'Bye, pee!' 99

66 Pretty soon you will be able to wear underpants and go pee on the potty, just like Mommy and Daddy. 99

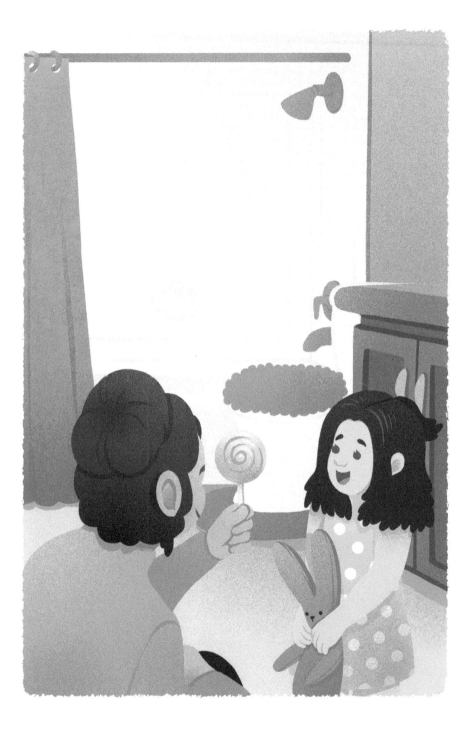

introduce the toilet

EVEN IF YOUR CHILD IS PARTIALLY FAMILIAR with the toilet, it's always a good idea to introduce him to it officially: That way his ideas about it come from you, not somewhere else. The more the child knows about the toilet and bathroom, the more comfortable he will be when training starts. For instance, "Little Bob, this is called the toilet or the potty. When you're a big boy, you sit on this to pee or poop instead of using a diaper. When you are all done, you flush the toilet, like this. It's not a toy, so we don't play with it."

saying hello

The first step in getting your child comfortable about the bathroom is to change her diapers in the bathroom instead of in her room or wherever else you have a changing area. You want your kiddo to start doing bathroom things in the bathroom, because that is what will be expected once you put her in underwear. Changing your child all over the house gives mixed signals. Once she feels comfortable being changed in the bathroom, it will be easier for her to feel comfortable sitting on the potty.

choose a reward

Finding the perfect reward is essential to your child's success with potty training. As with most people, children are more motivated when the situation directly benefits them. Most kids won't want to potty train just because you ask nicely!

So, to get your kiddo motivated, pick an immediately tangible reward. Telling Little Bob he will get a new bike or be able to pick out a new toy at the store *after* he learns to go pee on the potty is going to mean nothing to him. Kids need to be consistently rewarded every single time they are successful on the potty during training time for it to work.

I always tell parents to find a reward their child will really like. It can be anything, but I strongly hint at it being a candy treat. I know, I know . . . you're not supposed to reward children with food, and I completely understand this concept, but potty training will be so much easier if you do!

Toddlers aren't motivated by much else because their life experiences are limited, but boy do kids know which foods they like and do not like. That said, the reward could be anything *your child* finds to be a treat. I have used everything from M&M's to Goldfish to raisins . . . you want it to be small enough that you feel comfortable giving it to her many times throughout the day, yet satisfying enough to keep her willingly going to the bathroom all day.

I know there will be those parents who will try different rewards. I have had parents try a basket full of little toys as the reward—it just doesn't work. Kids may be excited about that little car for a few minutes, but after five or six new cars, the allure wears off. You will need to reward your child many, many times. There are instances when I have had kids successfully pee 15 to 20 times on the potty in ONE DAY . . . so, even if your child pees 5 times in a day, that equals 35 cars by the end of one week—and you need to continue the reward for at least two weeks. Just get a bag of M&M's!

Coupled with a food treat, I also use a sticker chart that I tape on the bathroom wall or door. Not all kids like stickers, but I find it's always worth a chance—that way he actually gets rewarded *twice* every time he goes to the bathroom. Trying to remove a sticker from its sheet is really good for a toddler's fine motor skills, so I allow him to pick a sticker, take it off, and put it on the chart himself. If Little Bob looks like he is struggling, ask him if he would like help: "If you want help, say, 'Help, please.'"

equipment

Things you will need:

- » A few new indoor activities (puzzles, coloring, Legos, etc.)
- » Overnight pull-ups, different from what the child currently wears
- » See-through jar to keep treats in
- » Several types of drink choices
- » Short shirt
- » Stepping stool for the toilet
- » Sticker chart
- » Stickers
- » Toilet trainer
- » Treats
- » Two or three packs of new underwear

For some reason the subject of a potty chair versus a toilet trainer has always been a hot topic at my potty-training workshops. From my experience, parents tend to gravitate toward buying the potty chair because it is cute and little—the perfect size for a toddler. Not only that, but it also comes in pretty colors and designs with favorite characters on it and makes cool noises when you "flush" it! I have very strong opinions on why I don't use potty chairs. I have actually stopped random people at the store from making that purchase, which I will continue to do every time I see it happening!

A toilet trainer or potty seat is a seat that fits on top of the *real* toilet and is the easiest and best way to potty train your child. This tool will help your child feel comfortable sitting up on the big toilet right from the start, instead of teaching her one procedure and then having to teach her another. When using a toilet trainer, it is important that your child can step up to the potty herself, which is why a step stool is required.

I do not, in any way, benefit from what I am about to tell you, but you need to know: The BabyBjörn toilet trainer is, hands down, the best one I have ever used. I require my clients to purchase one before I start helping them train, and, if they can't get one in time, I bring it to them—that's how great it is. The most common complaint I receive from parents about toilet trainers is that many are not secure on the toilet, which makes the child afraid to sit on it because she ends up sliding around. The BabyBjörn trainer eliminates that problem with a rubber bumper along the outside to prevent slipping. It also has a locking mechanism on the inside that will secure it to any toilet size or shape—I've yet to find a toilet it hasn't been able to fit onto. (That is not me challenging you to find one.)

why i don't use potty chairs

Sorry, but I'm going to give my little rant here.

Potty chairs are not real toilets, and they give the false idea that kids will be able to use that specific toilet every time they need to go to the bathroom.

Who wants a child to dump out her pee pot by herself? Because she will try.

A potty chair creates a fear of "the big potty" because your child won't be used to sitting up so high.

It also creates a fear of the flushing sound in public restrooms because your child is used to her potty making car revving noises, flashing lights, or playing ditties when it flushes.

You will have to transition her to the big toilet regardless. Why create extra steps?

Plus, cleaning poop out of the potty chair is traumatizing. Just, eewww.

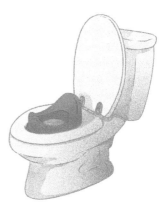

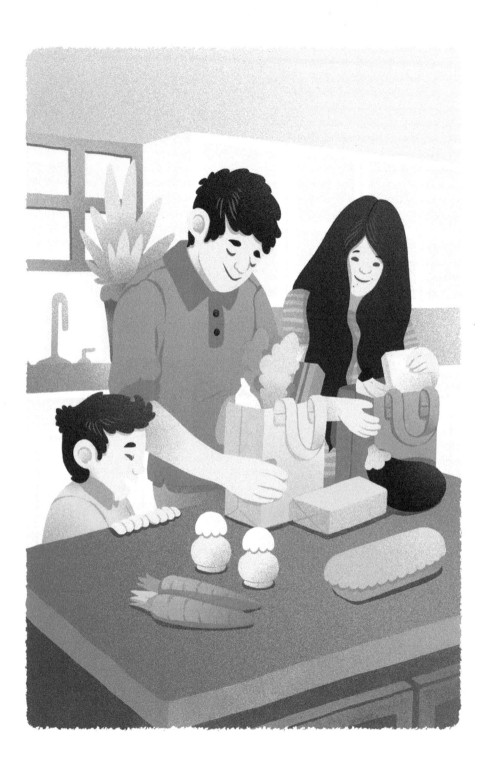

STEP 5:

prepare for the three days

ALL RIGHT, IT'S OFFICIALLY TIME TO TAKE THE LEAP. I want you to get out your calendars and choose *three* consecutive days for which you can honestly commit the full amount of time. Potty training is going to work only if you put in the effort and follow through until the end. *Trying it for half a day and letting your child decide she doesn't like it is not an option.*

it's not a game

Once, on a potty-training client intake form, a mom basically told me through several different answers that her child "didn't like it." So, that was the end of potty training. She didn't want to "play the game anymore" (a direct quote). Potty training isn't a game, and while you can make it *so* much fun and a memorable experience, you have to let your child know that once we take those diapers away, underwear is the new way of life.

I may sound harsh (and I am sorry if I come off that way), but I am trying to empower you. It is so easy to give in to what our children want, because what parent wants to see his or her child upset? Your kiddo will most likely cry during this process, but only because this will be new, and crying is one of the biggest ways children can let us know their feelings. But I can tell you, there is no greater feeling than the moment your child "gets it" and is so incredibly proud of herself.

That was a bit of a tangent, I know, but it's a point I cannot reiterate enough—and also the biggest reason parents fail at potty training: *Do not give in* to the crazy, unpredictable wants of your little human during this potty-training time. *No*, you can't have the whole bag of M&M's, and *no*, you may not have your diapers back!

choose the three days wisely

Pick three days and commit. I usually tell my clients to pick a long weekend when you have no other plans or commitments. You will literally be stuck in the house for the next two or three days straight. I mean it: no plans, conference calls, or quick e-mails. You should put your phone inside a cabinet and leave it there, because your eyes must be on your child 24/7, and cell phones are a parent's biggest distraction from their children; I'm guilty of this as well.

plan ahead

Once you have picked your three days (you have, right?), then it's time to start planning. *Yay!* Poop and pee—get excited!

Here are some things you should have planned and completed before you start your fun-filled (pee- and poop-filled) weekend:

GROCERIES: Breakfast, lunch, dinner, snacks, rewards, and, most importantly, several different types of drinks for your child.

(And also some wine or hard liquor for you. I won't judge you if you start drinking at noon . . . just kidding!) Oh, and make sure to have carpet cleaner or floor cleaner and lots of paper towels.

MEALS: You won't have time to cook because if you're cooking, your eyes aren't on your child. Buy salads and prepared meals, make meals ahead of time, or order in. It's just a few days; try to make it work. Hopefully, you will have some additional help at home during this time, so one person can cook while the other stays with the kid in underwear.

NEW ACTIVITIES: Consider puzzles, books, crayons, Play-Doh, and the like. You will be stuck in the house, so you don't want your child to feel stir-crazy. The way to fix that problem is to make sure she is never bored. Being able to divert your child's attention to new and exciting activities is going to save you. Things to keep in mind: You don't want new activities that are too messy because, at a moment's notice, she may start peeing. For that reason, you should also cross off using any dress-up clothes from your list of activities. Oh, and no new movies or anything like that; watching TV is, unfortunately, on the "no-no" list. I saved that for last—*yay, potty training!*

WORK: Please do not bring work home with you during this time. Trust me, I know it's hard, as I am currently working, taking care of my children full-time, and writing this book. It's so easy these days for our work lives and home lives to blend, but they just can't during your potty-training weekend. It's your child's time now, and work can wait. If it cannot, then choose a different time to start this process, because *you* aren't ready.

BABYSITTING HELP: If you have another child in the house, try to find some help during this time. The truth is, your eyes have to be on the child you are potty training nonstop, and your hands need to be free at a second's notice. If you are nursing or bottle-feeding a baby, you definitely won't be able to drop everything when Little Bob starts peeing on the floor. If you truly cannot find anyone to help you, then put up a baby gate in a safe room or set up a playpen where you are with your older child, because you will have to leave the younger child unattended at some point and you need the child to be safe while you are in the bathroom. Your potty-training child will have to come first during this time.

LOCATION: Please take my advice on this. Quarantine yourself during this time in an area of the house that is *very* close to a bathroom. When your child starts having an accident, you will need to pick her up and rush her to the bathroom. I'm fairly certain you don't want pee all up and down your house. If you have carpets, consider laying a plastic sheet or towels on the floor when your kiddo is playing.

I know this sounds exhausting and scary, but try to think of it as some really great bonding time with your child. Rediscover your house and engage with old toys in new ways; be silly and have a dance party. When you play with the toys alongside your child, she will become so much more engaged in the activity, and this potty-training time will be a more memorable experience for both of you.

make food your ally

In the spirit of making potty training as fun as possible, bring out the "fan favorites" at mealtime—those dishes your child really likes. As your focus must really be on potty training, the last thing you want to fight about is food.

Mealtimes are a "red flag" time of the day, which means kids often have accidents during this time. Because their food intake will be sporadic (they'll be drinking lots of fluids and getting rewards throughout the day), this is one reason I suggest buying food you know your child will eat.

The biggest thing to keep in mind is that you want your child to drink as much fluid as possible during these three days, so buy foods that encourage drinking.

FOODS THAT ENCOURAGE FLUID INTAKE

These aren't necessarily the best food choices, but, obviously, you can also feed your child healthy things in between some of these foods. These are just some types of food that will help you along this little journey.

- Applesauce
- Bread
- Chips
- Crackers
- Goldfish
- Hot dogs
- Peanut butter: apples with peanut butter, pb&j, spoonfuls, etc.
- Pizza
- Popcorn
- Watermelon

and, finally . . .

I find that parents completely stress out during this preparation time, more so than they tend to do during potty-training time. There is no need. You don't even realize it, but you are an *expert* at bathroom-related activities, so get confident. For example, you can pee on the potty and pull up your underwear like a boss, so take a deep breath, because you are going to be fine—and your kid is going to be fine, too.

But you won't be fine unless you read *all* of the next section ("During the Three Days") in advance! In this next section, I finally get to your burning question, "So what *am* I supposed to do?" Of course, I will continue to tell you more things not to do, but that's just because I have learned the hard way, and now I get to impart my shitty wisdom on you. (The puns never get old.)

during the three days

1 **ditch the diapers**

2 **start strong**

3 **drink, drink, drink**

4 **always be pottying**

5 **repeat**

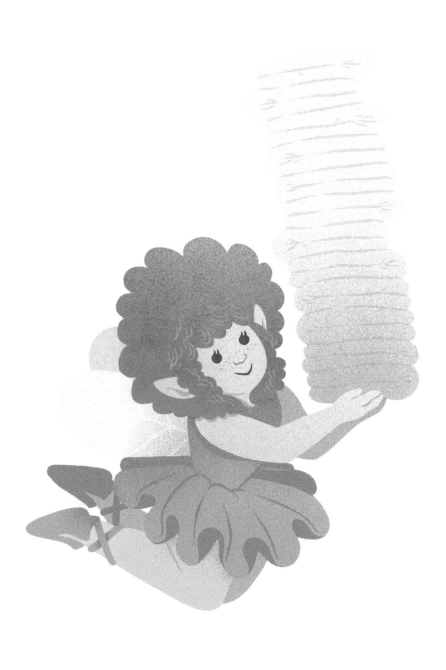

STEP 1:
ditch the diapers

BEFORE THE FIRST DAY OF POTTY TRAINING, you should already have talked this process over with your child thoroughly. This is a big milestone, and she deserves to know what is about to happen, why it is happening, how long it is going to happen, and how it benefits her. By now, your child should have seen her special toilet seat, her reward, and her new underwear. You should have built up this day so much that your child is now genuinely excited about it and is ready to tackle the challenge.

Alright, so my child wakes up at 7 a.m. I should start right away, right? No, definitely not. The most important thing in the morning is to get your child to eat a good breakfast. Oftentimes eating habits are a bit off during potty training because, as she learns to hold her bladder and bowels, she feels full inside and therefore won't eat as much. Mealtimes are also when kids tend to zone out—and then have accidents. So, it's best to let your child have one great meal and *then* start potty training.

First things first. It is time for the diapers to go buh-bye. Be happy because you are about to save so much money. Diapers cost more than $1,000 for a year's supply, whereas your new cost for overnight pull-ups (we will talk about this later) should be about $125 a year. Yay!

Grab a box or a bag and, together with your child, go around your house, collect all the diapers, and put them in the bag. Your child definitely needs to be part of this process, so make it a game. "Let's see if we can find all your diapers around the house as quickly as we can! I'll count!" Or, "We found some diapers. Can you throw them into the box?" If your child doesn't want to physically participate, that's okay—just make sure she sees you getting rid of all those diapers and understands that they really are going away *forever*.

Once you have collected diapers from *all* your secret hiding spots (don't forget the diaper bag or backpack), it's time to act like you are throwing them away or getting rid of them. I never actually recommend throwing away the diapers, because there are always diaper banks or other places you can donate unused diapers. If you don't know of any places in your area, please see my resource section (page 103) for suggestions.

Ways to ditch the diapers:

» Tell your child the mail carrier is going to take the diapers to other houses where babies need them. Put the box on your doorstep and, later on, have someone hide the box (when your child won't notice).

» Tell your child that the garbage collector is going to take them. Put all the diapers in a clean trash bag, and place the bag where the trash goes. Just make sure you move it later!

» Tell your child that the diaper fairy is going to deliver all those diapers to other little babies. Hide the bag of diapers in your closet or somewhere your child can't see them.

» If you have another baby in the house that needs the diapers, still box them all up, but make sure they are out of sight so they will be out of mind.

You get the idea, right? Your child has no diapers anymore. This whole process is important because if she asks for her diapers back, you can say, "What did we do with your diapers? We took all the diapers and we did [fill in the blank] with them. Now, other babies who need them have them. I am so proud of you for being such a big girl and wearing big-girl underwear!"

Your child needs to know that getting the diapers back isn't an option, and, because she was actually with you and helped you get rid of them, she knows this to be true . . . she just wanted to double-check to see if you were really serious about it.

QUICK FIX If at any point your child refers to herself as a baby or wants her diapers back because she is a baby, tell her she isn't a baby anymore, and you are so proud of her for being such a big kid. Sometimes not being the baby can be a hard transition, so just assure her that you love her a lot and it's exciting to grow up.

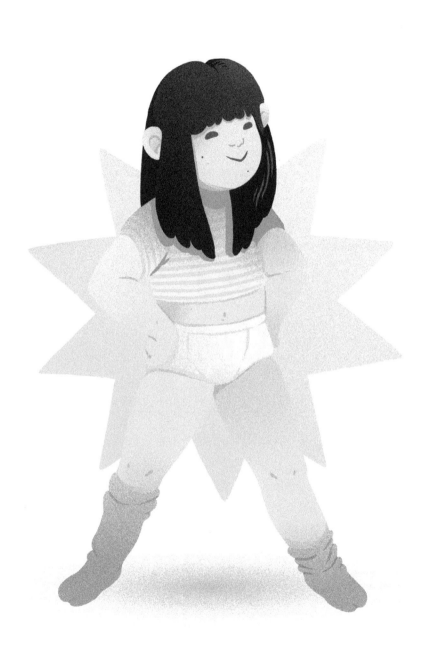

STEP 2:

start strong

THE LAST DIAPER TO GET RID OF is the one your child is currently wearing while collecting all the diapers around the house. You will walk with her to the bathroom, take off her diaper, and then put her in her new underwear. You will also put a short shirt on her. You want the shirt to be short enough so you can fully see her underwear. If the shirt hangs down to your child's knees, you won't be able to see when she starts peeing or if the underwear is damp. You also want to make things easy for you—so don't put pants on her. When she does have an accident, you definitely won't want those pants on her because that's one more thing you have to take off and wash. Taking off pants uses precious time you do not have when your child is peeing while you are holding her.

Next, show your kiddo her supplies and give her one last rundown of how this all will happen.

It's time for the serious training. You are going to follow your child around the house *all day*. Seriously, all day. The reason you must do this is that *catching your child's accident is absolutely the most essential part of the potty-training process*. When parents tell me their child continuously has accidents, the first question I ask is, "Where are you when she is having these accidents?" Almost always the answer is a variation of being in one room while the child is in

> **"** I am so proud of you for being such a big boy today, and now you get to wear big-kid underwear, like Mommy and Daddy. When you go pee on the potty, you get one treat and one sticker on your chart. When you go poop on the potty, you will get two treats and two stickers on your chart. It's really important that you tell Mommy (or whoever is doing the training) when you need to go potty. You need to keep your underwear dry and tell me when you need to go potty. **"**

another room, unattended. Your child has to be redirected every time she has an accident or she will never learn what she is supposed to do.

When you follow your child around the area of the house you have sequestered yourselves in, make sure you say to her every few minutes, "Tell me when you have to go potty." You will constantly repeat that statement throughout the day, and if you feel like you have said it too many times, you probably still haven't said it enough.

bathroom reminders

Do you notice the difference between "Tell me when you have to go potty" and "Do you want to go potty?" My questions (or statements) are firm, and the only choice you end up giving is whether she needs to go now or later, not if she *feels* like going at all. When you give affirming statements about how proud you are of her, you still subtly remind her about going to the bathroom. Sometimes it's a little bit of a mind game because you don't want to sound so incredibly redundant that your kid wants nothing to do with this, so change up the reminders.

- » "Tell me when you have to go potty."

- » "Is your underwear dry?"

- » "I am so proud of you for keeping your underwear dry right now."

- » "You're doing a great job of keeping your underwear dry today."

- » "I love how you're such a big boy today, and you're learning to go pee on the potty."

- » "Let me know when it's time to go potty."

- » "How many treats do you get when you put pee in the potty? You get one for peeing and two for pooping—that's so exciting!"

You can also do dry checks. Pat the underwear with the back of your hand to see if it is dry. If yes, draw attention to how great the child did keeping the underwear dry. Give her a high five or some physical recognition. If the underwear is damp, this is an opportunity to bring her to the bathroom, change her, and let her know she is supposed to keep the underwear dry. "Next time, tell me when you need to go potty." Hopefully, after doing this a few times, she can check her own underwear to see if it is wet or dry and then tell you.

When you know she should have to go soon say, "Soon we are going to sit on the potty to see if anything comes out."

If your child has a fun character on her underwear say, "Make sure you don't pee on Thomas the Tank Engine because that's yucky and Thomas won't like that."

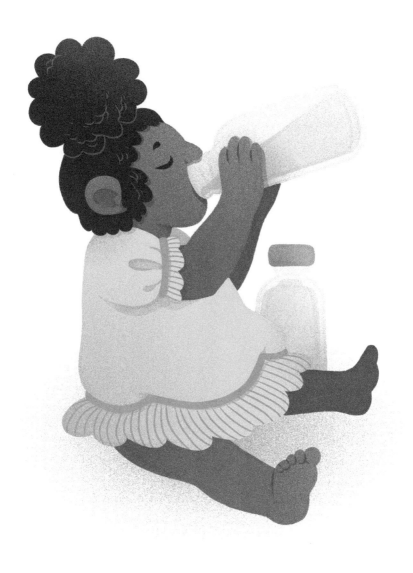

STEP 3:

drink, drink, drink

IT IS NOW TIME FOR YOUR CHILD TO PICK her drink of choice and drink it as quickly as possible. Your job for the next hour is to get your child to drink a lot of fluid, because the only way she will learn to pee on the potty is if she actually has to go to the bathroom. During training days you want to *increase* the amount of times she needs to go pee so she can practice her new bathroom procedures as many times as possible. You do that by filling her bladder. The child who pees eight times on the potty the first day is going to learn much more quickly than the child who pees on the potty only three times.

So why did I tell you to pick several different types of drinks for potty training? As every parent and caregiver knows, children are extremely fickle. One moment they love milk, and the next moment it's the worst thing they have ever tasted. Kids like choices, and they like to feel that they are in control. *Now* you can ask her which drink she would *like*. If she gets tired of that juice box, you can move along to the next drink choice. Keep rotating the drinks so she doesn't burn out drinking the same thing for days. You may have to get creative with ways to get your child to drink if she resists.

Are you a parent who doesn't allow your child to have juice? If yes, I am right there with you on that, but I urge parents to make an exception during potty training. Juice is loaded with sugar so I recommend you water it down before you give it to your child— especially if she never drinks it. If your child doesn't drink juice on a regular basis, she won't know you have watered it down, but it will be an exciting drink for her that, I bet, she will consume fairly quickly— and that's our goal.

Push the fluids really heavily during the first portion of the day and then taper off close to dinner. You want your child to have to go pee a lot during the day, but I promise you won't want her to wake up in the night having accidentally wet her bed because she went to bed with a really full bladder.

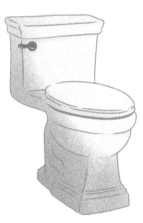

GET YOUR CHILD TO DRINK

» Take a sip of her drink first.
» Let her drink out of your cup.
» Tell your child you want to race to see who finishes the drink first.
» Use the "when/then" technique. "When you take three sips, then we can go play Legos!"

DRINK THIS

» Coconut water
» Decaffeinated tea
» Juice (watered down)

» Milk or chocolate milk
» Smoothies
» Water

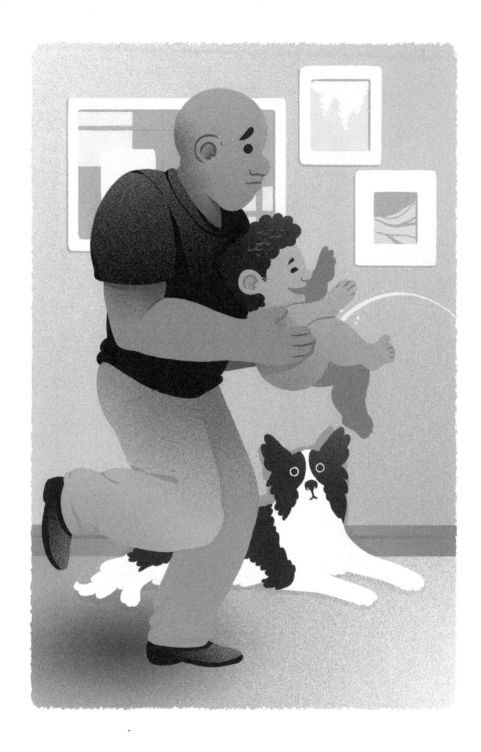

STEP 4:
always be pottying

AND NOW YOU WAIT. Your child shouldn't leave your eyesight *ever*. Wherever she goes, you go, reminding her every step of the way that she needs to tell you when she needs to go potty. In my opinion, this is the most stressful part of potty training: You have explained everything to your child and she hasn't had an accident yet, so you have no idea how she will respond and react. Usually, kids are completely surprised when pee starts running down their legs, especially if they have never worn underwear before—but you never know until it happens the first time.

As the saying goes, "accidents happen." Trust me, accidents will happen. The first couple of accidents are the most important, and they tell you a lot about your child. It is important to know how long she can hold her bladder and what kind of body cues she exhibits before, during, and after the accident. It is perfectly okay to keep a little notebook with you to jot down notes about pottying times. I do that. You think you can remember, but, after a little while, every bathroom trip blends into the other and they become a blur. If you know the last time she peed, when she drank fluid, and how long she can hold her bladder, you can stay one step ahead of your child by estimating the next time she should have to pee. After a couple of accidents, you will start to see a pattern to how long your child can "hold it."

If your child is consistently holding it for an hour and a half, you don't need to give as many bathroom reminders during the first 45 minutes after she uses the bathroom. Do start to give extra reminders, though, during the last 30 minutes of that time frame. And as I mentioned previously, you want your child to experience having a full bladder, which is why using a timer method isn't very effective.

that first accident

When your child starts to have her first accident, pick her up *mid-pee*! Carry her to the bathroom saying, "Oh no, pee goes in the potty, not on the floor," and then, as quickly as possible, get the underwear down and sit her on the potty. Be forewarned: You will probably get pee on yourself at some point. It's sterile, so don't worry about the pee puddle on the floor right now. The most important thing is to teach your child what to do in the bathroom. The floor can be cleaned later.

If you caught the accident quickly enough, you probably scared her when you picked her up, which means she probably stopped peeing and still has a half-full bladder. If this is the case, there is a chance that when you sit your child on the toilet, more pee will come out. If nothing comes out, she either emptied her bladder on the floor or is holding it and will have to pee again in another five minutes or so.

Regardless, praise your child up and down for sitting on the potty. Basically, overpraise your child for all the big-kid things he is doing this weekend—even if it is something small. "Wow, look at you!

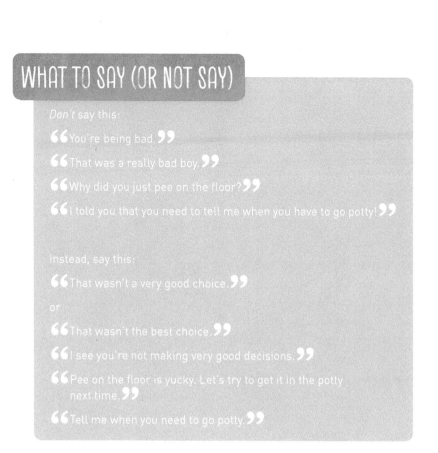

WHAT TO SAY (OR NOT SAY)

Don't say this:

"You're being bad."

"That was a really bad boy."

"Why did you just pee on the floor?"

"I told you that you need to tell me when you have to go potty!"

Instead, say this:

"That wasn't a very good choice."

or

"That wasn't the best choice."

"I see you're not making very good decisions."

"Pee on the floor is yucky. Let's try to get it in the potty next time."

"Tell me when you need to go potty."

You are such a big boy! Thank you for sitting on the potty so nicely, Little Bob." If he kicks and screams but has sat on that toilet even for one second, say, "Thank you for sitting on the potty. That was a good choice."

It's really important to be positive before you redirect your child. After she is done on the toilet, take some time to talk with her about the accident. Show her the dirty underwear and say, "Yucky, your underwear isn't dry anymore. We need to make sure it stays dry. Next time tell Mommy when you need to go potty." Then, with your child, walk over to where she peed on the floor and say, "This is really yucky. Your pee went on the floor instead of in the toilet. It's very important to tell Mommy when you need to go potty."

Now you can clean it up.

If your child doesn't know the difference between wet and dry yet, wet some underwear in the sink and let her feel the difference between wet underwear and dry underwear. "Do you feel how this underwear is wet and yucky? Feel this one—it's nice, clean, and dry. Let's try to keep your underwear nice and dry today."

after the first accident

Five minutes after the first accident, walk your child back to the bathroom and have her sit on the potty again. I do this because, usually, that first time is a bit traumatic. Things are calmer now, and she may still have to pee more. Have her sit on the potty *no longer than* one minute. Having your child sit on the potty for extended periods of time can be very distressing and can cause her to fear having to go to the bathroom. If your child is squirmy and needs to sit a bit longer, sing a song, such as "ABCs" or "Twinkle, Twinkle, Little Star," and she will usually calm down.

Even if she hasn't peed, take her off the potty, thank her for sitting so nicely, and give her *one* treat. *This is absolutely the only time I give a child a treat without any progress on the potty*. The reason I do this is because telling a child she will get something after she pees isn't the same as actually experiencing it firsthand. Once she receives the treat, she will understand what she is working for. Remind her that every time she puts pee in the potty, she will get one treat. *And* if she poops in the potty, she will get two treats.

what deserves a treat?

If at any point you see signs that your child has to go to the bathroom, have her go sit on the potty. If she says she doesn't have to go, you say, "When you [fill in the blank] (touch your underwear, grab yourself, etc.,) your body is showing me you have to go to the bathroom. Let's go sit on the potty and see if anything comes out. If you get any pee in the potty, you will get a treat!"

If she really doesn't want to go to the bathroom and you know for sure she needs to go, use the "when/then" technique. This usually works well because you get your child excited about something she will do after sitting on the potty, which encourages her to sit on the potty first. For example, "*When* you sit on the potty, *then* we can go play with your new blocks!" "*When* you put pee in the potty, *then* we can have Popsicles!" It's important to stay firm—the child needs to sit on the potty before she can do whatever you promised.

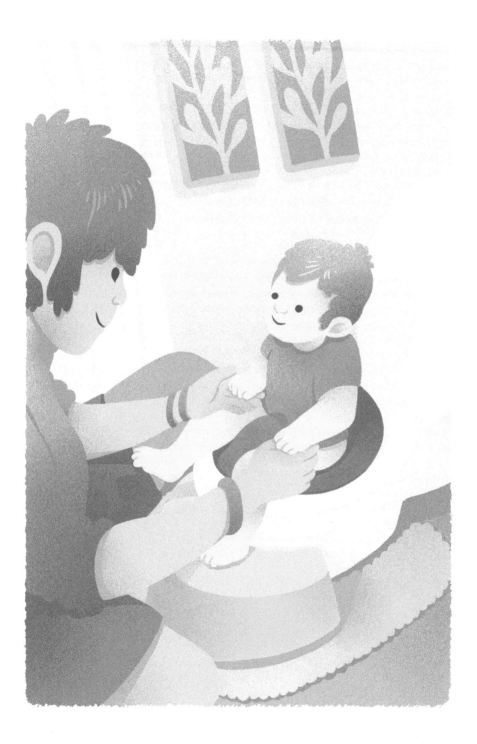

STEP 5:
repeat

YOU WILL REPEAT THESE FOUR STEPS during the three days of potty training. I know it seems like a lot, but you have to put in this heavy amount of work for only a short period of time compared to the rest of your child's life. If you don't hit it hard in the beginning, potty training can actually take a lot longer. It's worth this initial effort.

There will also be certain times of the day or common transitions when you will have your child sit on the potty to try to go, which really should help keep the random accidents at bay. Her body will start to respond to the new peeing schedule you have given her, and soon it will be normal to go to the bathroom during these times.

wearing pants and going outside

Depending on your child's progress, you can start adding more layers to the potty-training process, such as putting your child in pants or letting her play outside for a few minutes.

I generally put pants on kids toward the end of Day 2 or on Day 3. Pants add a challenge—not only because they are an extra layer to

PUT THE KIDDO ON THE POTTY

These are the most important times to sit your child on the toilet:

» When you arrive at a public place
» When you drop your child off at school
» Before and after mealtimes
» Before bath time
» Before going to sleep
» Before leaving the house
» Upon waking

remove when your child has to pee, but also because they hinder you from seeing your child's accident immediately. Usually you will notice the pants dampen when it's a bit too late and the accident is finished.

If your child has been fairly successful up to the middle of Day 2, let your kiddo play outside for a few minutes (15 to 20 minutes). This is usually a great reward after she has gone potty, and you will know she will be able to hold it for at least 30 minutes. *Do not do this on Day 1.* No matter what, your child's potty-training skills won't be developed enough on the first day to warrant playing outside far from the potty. Not only that, but on Day 1, you really don't know your child's body cues very well. It's best to play inside for the entire first training day.

Once outside, your child will likely want to stay outside. To prevent a potential tantrum, tell your child how much time she can have outside and then set a timer. Let her know every five minutes or so how much time is left to play outside. When the timer goes off, it won't be a complete surprise.

and whatever you do, *don't* do this

I have mentioned some things I recommend you plan ahead for, and a few things not to do, such as work from home during potty training or leave the house with your child during this time. I do have a few more things to add to the "no-no" list during this weekend, so get ready.

DO *NOT* LET YOUR CHILD WATCH TV OR PLAY ON THE IPAD. This might be a hard rule to follow, but every parent knows when children sit in front of the TV or an electronic device, they turn into little zombies. How many times do you have to say her name before your child responds to you? Zoning out usually means having an accident. A few successful pees in the potty do not make her an expert or mean the new procedures have been reinforced enough that peeing on the potty is now a habit. Kids forget because their conscious minds are basically turned off when the TV is turned on. If watching TV and playing with the iPad are a must for your child, then place her on a towel, sit next to her, and remind her every minute to tell you when she has to go to the bathroom.

DO NOT STARE AT YOUR PHONE FOR LONGER THAN 15 TO 30 SECONDS. Remember when I said your kids know how to manipulate you? Well, I promise they will have their pee accidents the exact second you are not paying attention or have left the room. The times when your child has to go pee are the only learning opportunities. If you miss those opportunities because you were playing Candy Crush, you'll have to pump your child full of fluids again, then wait until the next time she has to go to the bathroom. Bummer.

DO NOT LEAVE YOUR CHILD ALONE IN A ROOM. Once you put your child into underwear on Day 1 of training, you will be glued to your child until he goes to sleep—whether that's naptime or bedtime. If you go to the kitchen to get lunch, Little Bob is coming with you. If you have to go to the bathroom, Little Bob is coming, too. If you go to your room to change clothes because you got peed on, Little Bob comes along. If you have to put a load of pee underwear in the washer, Little Bob? Yes, he comes, too. Do you see the pattern? You have to be right there to catch every single accident your child has, or this won't work.

DO NOT GIVE BACK YOUR CHILD'S DIAPERS. If you give back your child's diapers because she demands them or throws a fit, you not only show your child she has complete power, but you also set yourself up to fail when you decide to potty train for real in the future. If you give the diapers back once, your child will expect them back every time and will not take you seriously when you say it's time to ditch the diapers. Usually a power struggle will ensue, and your child will throw the tantrum of a lifetime.

Two examples come to mind here, both with girls who had tried potty training in the past, but for which the parents reacted differently in each situation. One mom, a psychologist, wanted to bargain with her child during her screaming fit about wanting diapers back. She refused to put underwear on her daughter or continue potty training until they could talk it through thoroughly. The other mom was a stay-at-home mom who, during her daughter's tantrum (because the child didn't want to put underwear on and wanted her diaper), somehow managed to get the underwear on the screaming girl. Only one of these little girls ended up potty trained. I will let you guess which one. (Okay, I'll tell you! The psychologist's daughter got her diapers back, and it took another six months to get her potty trained.) Don't do it.

DO NOT *ASK* IF SHE *WANTS TO* OR *NEEDS TO* GO TO THE BATHROOM.
Honestly, this is one of my biggest tricks with potty training. It seems so simple, but you will be amazed how hard it is to keep from asking your child if she wants to, or has to, go to the bathroom.

Asking your child, "Do you *want* to go potty?" allows the option to say "no." But really, there is no choice anymore. You've put her in underwear, so she needs to pee on the potty—no choice about it. And really, who *wants* to go to the bathroom? Even adults are annoyed by the task, yet we have to do it. If your child is in the middle of playing with a toy or doing something fun, she is *never* going to want to stop and go to the bathroom if you give her a choice. *Never.*

If you *ask* your child, "Do you *need* to go potty?" she really can't answer that honestly, so she will automatically tell you "no." Her little kidneys make about 10 drops of urine per minute, so really she could trickle out some pee whenever she sits down to try—kids just don't know that yet.

Instead of asking, replace the questions with the statement, *"Tell me when you need to go potty."* When you say this, it doesn't really require a response from your child, but she still hears the information and can now think about it and cue you when she needs to go.

I swear this works.

DO NOT EXPECT YOUR CHILD TO TELL YOU SHE HAS TO GO *BEFORE* SHE STARTS PEEING. Okay, so now you know to say, "Tell me when you have to go potty." Realize, however, she isn't going to come right out and tell you ahead of time—for a while. As I said before, you are teaching a new habit and procedure. Your child is learning about her body. Once she grasps the concept and feels confident, she will be able to tell you when she needs to go. Some kids do this two days after they start training, and others do this a week or two after starting.

DO NOT SHOW FRUSTRATION OR ANGER. Do not put your child into timeout or reprimand her for having an accident. It's really important to keep potty training as light and fun as possible. If you get angry with your child on a regular basis while in the bathroom, she will start to think you're always going to be angry in there. Fake it till you make it! Think about something happy, like the drink(s) you're going to have with (or instead of) dinner.

DO NOT GIVE YOUR CHILD HER REWARD UNLESS SHE IS SUCCESSFUL ON THE POTTY. I like to keep a child's reward in a glass jar on the middle of the counter where it can be seen. It's good for her to be reminded visually that she, too, benefits from this whole fiasco. There will be times when your child will see her treat and demand it. That's the time you firmly ask, "How can you get one of these?" If she doesn't answer, remind her that peeing on the potty will get her one and pooping on the potty will get her two. Stick to your guns, because if you give her a treat whenever, then she won't have any motivation to go use the toilet. You've already given her the treat, so what's the point?

DO NOT LET YOUR CHILD TELL YOU "NO." There will be many times when you will have to give your child bathroom reminders or encourage her to go. You may, at some point, get a little pushback—usually in the form of a fit or a flat-out "no." If she does say "no," firmly respond, "Please do not tell me 'no.' Peeing in your underwear isn't a choice." Or, "Please do not tell me 'no.' You have to tell me when you need to go potty."

If your child throws a fit, try to push through it because, usually, it's just a stage to try to gain some control over the situation. If she has an accident, carry her to the bathroom (kicking and screaming and all), take off the wet underpants, and sit her on the potty. Try to keep her on the potty by distracting her with a song or telling her what a good job she is doing sitting on the potty.

DON'T DO THIS

» Do not *ask* if she has to or wants to go to the bathroom.
» Do not expect your child to tell you *before* she has to pee (at the beginning).
» Do not give back your child's diapers.
» Do not give her a reward unless she is successful on the toilet.
» Do not leave your child alone in a room.
» Do not let her tell you "no."
» Do not let your child watch TV or play on electronic devices.
» Do not show anger or frustration with your child.
» Do not use your phone for more than 15 to 30 seconds at a time.

If that doesn't work and the tantrum continues, take her off the toilet, *thank* her for sitting on the potty, and tell her, "We will try again later." Once she is cleaned up and completely calm from her fit, tell her that behavior is not okay and that next time she has to tell you when she needs to go potty. It's appropriate for your child to apologize for throwing a tantrum. Give her a big hug, tell her how proud you are of her for being such a big kid today, and acknowledge how hard it can be. It's nice to be validated sometimes.

If your child throws a fit over something nontoilet related, just let her. Do not try to rationalize or bribe the child. Sit calmly next to her while she's throwing her fit, and once she starts to calm down, try to divert her attention to something new, such as an activity you can do together. Even if she doesn't want to play, if you start playing and acting like it's *so* much fun, chances are she will come over and join you. Tantrum over.

after
the
three
days

1 **always be celebrating**

2 **family members and other caregivers**

3 **naptime and nighttime**

4 **accidents**

5 **keep teaching**

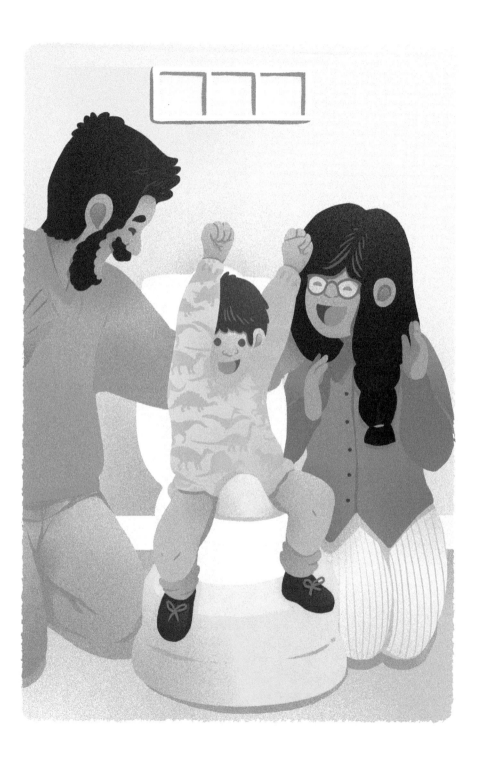

STEP 1:
always be celebrating

YOU'VE PASSED THE FIRST THREE DAYS of potty training. Congratulations! Keep celebrating and rewarding your child. You may be tired of pretending to be as excited about pee as you would be about winning the lottery, but trust me, your child isn't tired of it.

Because you still want your child to feel motivated to use the bathroom, it's best to wean her gradually from the attention and rewards instead of cutting her off completely at once. Usually the sticker chart will be the first reward to go because she will start to forget about it. Keep the sticker chart up for the initial three days, and when your child starts forgetting about it, stop reminding her.

Since the food treat is usually the key motivating factor to potty training, continue to give it to your child for at least two weeks—and even longer for pooping on the potty. If after two weeks you feel your child really has the hang of peeing on the potty, stop giving her a treat if she forgets to ask for it. Your child may remember a couple of times, which is okay, but after two days, you should say, "I'm so proud of you for being such a big kid. You get two treats for pooping on the potty, and that's how you can get treats now. Please tell me when you have to go potty."

There is a chance your child may regress a bit when you do this. It's important to stay firm. If she has an accident, do as you have been doing—run her to the bathroom. After she is done and cleaned up, say, "You know peeing in your underwear isn't a choice anymore. You have to tell me when you need to go potty." If she doesn't start making the right choice for a day or two, bring the reward back, but *only* reward her when she remembers. Do not continue this for more than a month because, if it goes on much longer, the treat will become a behavioral issue, not a potty-training issue.

family members and other caregivers

ONE WAY TO CONFUSE YOUR CHILD and make the potty-training process take even longer is by not having everyone who takes care of your child on the same page. If you have gotten this far in the book, you are most likely choosing this method to use when potty training your child. Any person who is with your child in the bathroom should become knowledgeable about this plan. I have seen more than one argument between parents when one has read the plan and the other parent clearly has not. Don't let that be you.

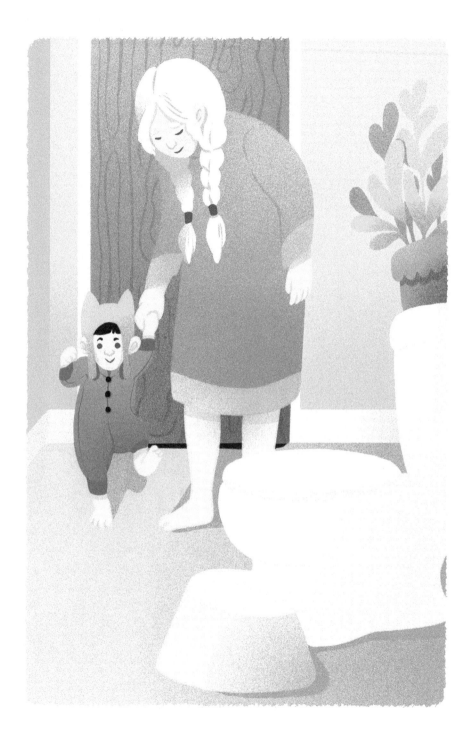

partner up

Communicate with your partner. If you have been the one potty training your child at home, then you will know your child's cues and have a whole method down with her in the bathroom. Your partner may not have had as many opportunities to be involved with the process. Be patient. If your partner is keeping an eye on the child while you shower or run errands, explain the specific things to look for when your child might have to go to the bathroom, and some things to avoid, such as letting her watch TV or play on the iPad.

at school

Your child's teacher will be willing to help as much as possible and should be a great part of your support system, but unless the school has a potty-training program, it is not the teacher's job to potty train your child. Let the teacher know the best way to support your child during the school day, but if there are too many accidents at school, the teacher will, most likely, tell you your child needs to go back to wearing diapers when not at home—which will just confuse and hinder your kiddo during training. It will take time for your child to get used to going to the bathroom in a different place, with a different person, and with different procedures, so let your child's teacher know what kinds of things to do or say to help your child keep her underwear dry.

Talk with your child about going to the bathroom at school before you send him back. For example, "Little Bob, you have done such a good job going pee and poop on the potty at home; now you will use the potty at school, too. At home you tell Mommy when you need to go potty, and at school you will tell your teacher." Before you leave the child for the day, it helps to have a conversation among the three of you so your child knows he is supported by both of you in the same way.

One good rule of thumb is to bring your child to the bathroom she will use at school as soon as you drop her off. Doing this gives her the chance to go to the bathroom with you, the person she's most comfortable with, and this, in turn, will make her feel more comfortable using the school's bathroom. Not only that, but knowing she has emptied her bladder at the beginning of the school day means she should be able to stay dry for a couple of hours, which helps the teacher know when to start giving your child extra bathroom reminders. You should also get into the habit to having her go right before leaving school, as well; that way you have the car ride covered, too.

everywhere else

It's always a good habit to bring a newly potty-trained kid to the bathroom immediately upon arriving at any new location. Nothing is worse than getting halfway through with grocery shopping, only to have your child tell you she needs to go to the bathroom.

FIVE TIPS FOR CAREGIVERS WHO AREN'T YOU

If you can't get your partner or other caregivers to read this plan, these are the five most important things they should know.

1. Do not *ask* the child if she wants/needs to go to the bathroom: "*Tell me* when you need to go."
2. Do not leave the child alone in a room.
3. Be present for each accident so you can redirect the child in the middle of her accident instead of after the accident.
4. Give rewards and praise for every time she successfully goes potty.
5. Do not show anger or frustration.

naptime and nighttime

THE KEYS TO STAYING DRY AT NIGHT are an empty bladder and no fluids two hours before bedtime!

The *only* time I use pull-ups during potty training is while a child is sleeping, and I usually recommend using nighttime pull-ups, which *are* different than regular pull-ups. Most likely you haven't used these with your child before, so they should look different than the regular diapers or pull-ups worn previously. I know, telling you it's okay to use pull-ups seems contradictory to what I said earlier, but I find it extremely unfair to expect a two- to three-year-old to stay completely dry during training, especially if she cannot get up to use the bathroom herself in the night.

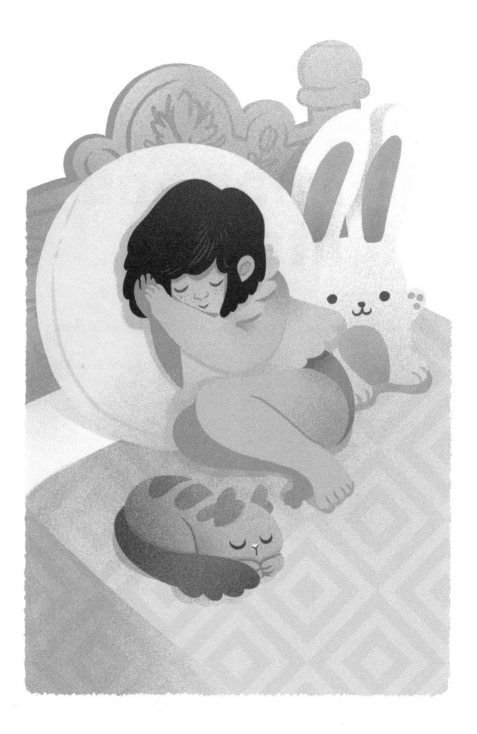

So, here are my tricks for continued success:

1. CALL THESE PULL-UPS "SLEEPING UNDERWEAR."
   That way your child still believes they are related to underwear.

2. THE SLEEPING UNDERWEAR GOES ON RIGHT BEFORE GETTING INTO BED.
   Do not let your child walk around the house while wearing it—
   that is basically like wearing diapers, which is the opposite of
   what we are trying to accomplish here.

3. THE SLEEPING UNDERWEAR COMES OFF IMMEDIATELY UPON WAKING.
   Well, within a minute or so. You don't want to give your child
   enough time to wake up and pee in it.

4. YOUR CHILD'S REGULAR UNDERWEAR MUST GO ON TOP OF THE
   SLEEPING UNDERWEAR—EVERY TIME.
   When your child looks down, she should see underwear. This is
   a mind trick. Your child has been trained to use the bathroom
   while in her underwear, and for the most part, she will continue
   to do so even while sleeping. Of course accidents happen and
   bladders need time to train.

If your child still takes a nap (wow, you are so lucky!), this will be
the testing ground to see how well she can control her bladder while
sleeping. Kids are able to keep themselves dry for a nap way before
they are able to stay dry all night—naps are much shorter.

an empty bladder

To set your child up for overnight success, it's extremely important that she goes to the bathroom before going to sleep, whatever time of day that is. If your child goes to sleep with a full bladder, she'll absolutely wet the bed. She just can't help it.

A little trick I do at night is have kids go to the bathroom 30 minutes before bedtime, and then one more time as the very last thing they do before hopping into bed. That way, they have had two chances to empty their bladders, which are now, most likely, completely empty.

Expect that your child will have to go to the bathroom each time she wakes up. So, after a minute or so, walk her to the bathroom so she can sit down to try. This is also the time to take off the "sleeping underwear" so she doesn't get the chance to walk around the house wearing it.

QUICK FIX If your child resists taking off his "sleeping underwear," say, "This is your sleeping underwear, and, since you aren't sleeping right now, you need to take it off." Once you get it off, say, "Thank you for being such a big boy and taking off your sleeping underwear."

Your child no longer needs sleeping underwear when she has been able to remain dry for five to seven nights. At that point, you can attempt to have her sleep with only her regular underwear and see how it goes. If she has an accident, it's okay to put her back into the sleeping underwear. Remember, at night it really *is* an accident.

no fluids before bedtime

Nighttime fluids are always a touchy subject with parents; many who come to me still give their kids sippy cups filled with milk before bed to keep the child's belly full overnight. They are often afraid that cutting back on the milk may disrupt the child's sleeping patterns, but there are other ways to fill a kid's belly before bedtime.

Nutritionist and colleague Allison Reyna suggests these options as healthy choices that will curb your child's appetite until morning:

» Apple or pear slices

» Applesauce

» Cheese sticks

» Hard-boiled eggs

» Plain yogurt with fruit and a squirt of honey

» Whole-grain pita and hummus

If you do give your child a large amount of fluid before bed, gradually start to wean it away instead of stopping cold turkey. If you give Little Bob eight ounces of milk before bed, give him seven ounces tomorrow, and then six ounces the next night, and so on, until there is no more milk to be given. Let your child know why you are doing this. For example, "Little Bob, now that you are such a big boy and go pee on the potty, I have to help you keep your underwear dry at night. If you drink too much milk, you will have to go potty when you are sleeping, and we want you to go potty when you are awake."

From years of field experience, I know kids often pee in their sleeping underwear or have an accident in the morning when they first stir. One way to keep your child from doing that is to get her up before she is awake enough to pee in her bed. For example, if your child consistently wakes up at 7 a.m., set your alarm for 6:45 a.m., get her up a little early, and take her to the bathroom. You can then train her bladder by waking her up one minute later every morning until you have reached her normal wake-up time.

Most of the time, when her body is ready, your child will start staying dry overnight all on her own. The little 21-month-old I potty trained was keeping herself dry overnight at two and a half, while her twin brother didn't stay dry until after he turned four. Each child develops differently, and staying dry isn't really something you can force. It will happen when the bladder is more developed.

QUICK FIX If your child has an accident during the night and is woken by it, most likely she went to bed with an extremely full bladder. Either give her less fluid or wait to put her to bed until after she has gone pee on the potty.

Be patient with your child during this overnight process. Each child develops differently, so make sure your child knows there is no shame in having an overnight accident.

accidents

NO ONE WANTS THEIR CHILD TO BACKSLIDE with potty training less than I do. It makes me look bad. However, there are some extenuating circumstances that may cause some potty-training troubles, such as:

- » A new sibling
- » Changing schools
- » Family traveling
- » Illness
- » Moving

- » Nightmares
- » Parents traveling
- » Switching teachers
- » Stressful events

So . . . just avoid those things, mmmkay? The most important thing is not to get angry or upset at your child if accidents happen. There is *always* a reason a child has an accident—whether you weren't paying attention to the warning signs, she didn't want to stop playing with her toys, or there was a new teacher at school she didn't feel comfortable enough with to tell when she needed to go to the bathroom. If you can pinpoint the reason behind your child's accidents, you can find other ways to support her and get her back on track.

One trick to be aware of is your child using bathroom-related things to manipulate you—for example, coming out of the bedroom soon after being put to bed because she "has to go potty." One hundred percent of the time parents fall for this. (You had her go pee

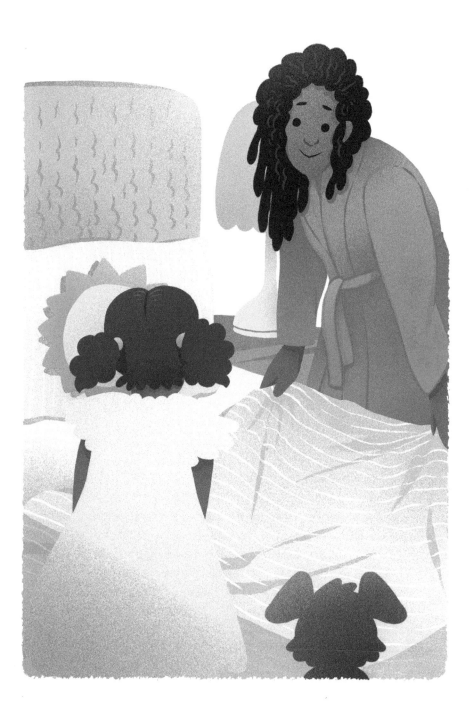

immediately before she got into bed, right?) If you know she peed five minutes ago, then you will know she is playing you. If you realize you forgot to have her sit on the potty before going to bed, then her potty plea may be legit. Accompany her to the bathroom either way, so you know if she really did need to go. If nothing comes out, tell her you know she didn't actually have to go, and next time will be different.

quick answers to common questions

Q: WHAT DO I DO WHEN MY KID HAS AN ACCIDENT?

A: First, stay calm, which I know is hard to do, especially when you thought your child had this potty-training thing in the bag. If you are at home, treat the accident just like you would have when you were potty training. Scoop up your child mid-pee and redirect him to the bathroom as quickly as possible. Then say (without anger or frustration), "Little Bob, you are supposed to tell me when you need to go potty. Did you forget? Now your underwear and your pants are very wet and yucky. You have to tell me every time you need to go potty, because peeing on the floor isn't a choice. Your pee always needs to go in the potty, okay? Let's go clean up the pee that went onto the floor instead of inside the potty."

If you are out in public, I'm very, very sorry. Even though accidents in public are embarrassing for everyone involved, it bothers me when people tell their kids, "It's okay. Accidents happen." Yes, accidents happen, like spilling the box of cereal on the floor or dropping a cup of milk, and those are okay. It shouldn't, at this point, be okay if your child pees anywhere else but the toilet, and you can let her know this by being firm without yelling or getting angry. If you just tell her "It's okay" every time, then you are literally saying it's okay to do this! It's not okay!

You can say, "Oh no, you peed on the floor at [fill in the blank]. I don't have extra clothes for you now, so your underwear is going to be wet until we get home, and then you can put on clean, dry underwear. You need to tell me every time you have to go potty, even when we're not home, so I can help you avoid accidents like this." There are consequences to actions, so this is a lesson to be learned.

Q: WHAT DO I DO IF MY CHILD STARTS TO BACKSLIDE INTO BAD HABITS?

A: No offense, but if your child starts backsliding into bad habits, it is most likely because you have become lax about whatever that new bad habit is. For instance, your child refusing to wash her hands because you haven't really made her do it, or crying and throwing a tantrum on Monday morning when you take off her sleeping underwear because someone let her run around the house with it on for too long the day before.

Bad habits are most likely a behavioral problem that can be fixed with a little extra reinforcement. If you want to break a habit, address it every single time you see it happening, or it will never change. We correct our children's speech when they use the past tense of a word incorrectly, and eventually they learn the correct word. If you correct your child's negative behavior each time you see it, she will start to learn a new positive behavior instead.

Q: WHAT SHOULD I DO IF MY CHILD STARTS WETTING THE BED?

A: There are a few different reasons children wet the bed, including:

- Being constipated
- Being sick
- Having poor muscle tone in the pelvic floor
- Having too much fluid before bed
- Not using the toilet right before bed
- Stressful events
- Sexual or physical abuse

If your child wets the bed, your first step is to figure out the reason behind it; otherwise, you will have a hard time helping her avoid this in the future.

If you have an older child who wets the bed, have her seen by your doctor. It isn't common knowledge that constipation is a significant cause of bed-wetting, and even though your child may be pooping regularly, there can still be a large backup in the intestines. I will address constipation more in my poop section (see page 99).

Q: WHAT IS MY NEXT STEP IF THE INITIAL THREE DAYS OF POTTY TRAINING DIDN'T WORK?

A: As I have said before, persist with this plan for at least 10 days before stopping. While three days is long enough to introduce something new, it definitely isn't long enough to create a new habit for your child, especially when she has had three years of peeing in a diaper and only three days of peeing on the potty. Try to maintain perspective on that point.

Q: WHAT IF MY CHILD IS BEING STUBBORN AND UNCOOPERATIVE?

A: If your child is being uncooperative, this is most likely a behavioral issue and not a sign that she isn't ready for potty training. My most difficult child threw screaming tantrums for the first two days of potty training, with little pottying success, because she was the boss of the house. She couldn't control this situation, so she tested her mom's limits in every way possible. I've never been more proud of a mom than I was of this one because she pushed through, and even though it took her a little longer than the three-day period to get her daughter trained (in this case, six days), it worked, and she was amazed at the change in her daughter's behavior.

Q: WHAT SHOULD I SAY TO MY CHILD IF SHE TELLS ME SHE IS SCARED OF THE POTTY?

A: I've come across children who are genuinely scared of or intimidated by the potty and also children who use "I'm scared" as a tactic to avoid doing things they don't want to do.

When a child says she is scared, most parents will coddle her and say something like, "It's okay, you don't have to do it if you're scared," instead of saying, "It's okay to be scared, but being scared shouldn't keep us from trying new things."

If you think your child is genuinely intimidated by the potty, it's most likely because it's bigger than she is, she isn't really sure what it is, it makes loud noises, and she has no personal experience with it. For these reasons, I encourage people to introduce the toilet to their kiddos and explain that it isn't something to be scared of. Allowing your child to flush toilet paper down or flush after you have used the toilet are good ways to get her to feel more comfortable before you start potty training.

Q: WHAT SHOULD I DO IF MY CHILD HAS ACCIDENTS WHEN MY PARTNER IS IN CHARGE, BUT HAS NO ACCIDENTS WHEN WITH ME?

A: If this happens, then your partner—not your child—is doing something wrong. You know your child can go to the bathroom perfectly fine with you. Ask your partner for an honest answer to the question: "What were *you* were doing when our kiddo had her accident?" Most of the time, this will explain everything! Almost always it involves a mind occupied elsewhere or being in a different room.

Q: IT HAS BEEN 10 DAYS, AND THIS PLAN WAS A COMPLETE DISASTER. WHAT SHOULD I DO?

A: If this plan really didn't work and you had hardly any (if any) progress, contact me for further help. I always have clients complete an extensive intake form so I can easily pinpoint any red flags, and then I coach them over the phone or e-mail or provide in-home support.

I have a 98.5 percent success rate with children I have personally potty trained, which doesn't take into account people I have helped along the way in my workshops or in other ways. If this plan didn't work, there is definitely a reason (or reasons), and I can help you figure that out.

hey, what about poop?

I briefly addressed how it's important for your child to have poops that aren't hard before you start potty training, but other than that I haven't really mentioned it. Pooping on the potty can be a completely different battle than peeing on the potty—especially if your child is constipated. Poop is the one thing a kid can control and hold, and hold, and hold, which creates a really shitty situation! Your child can actually be pooping on a regular basis without you even knowing she is backed up inside her little body. If your child is constipated, she will have a hard time with potty training because her engorged rectum is pushing up against her bladder, causing pee to spill out in frequent accidents.

Here are some symptoms and signs that your child may be constipated:

» Bed-wetting and frequent peeing accidents

» Frequent, mad dashes to the bathroom to pee

» Infrequent or irregular pooping

» Holding poop in (by crossing her legs tightly, hiding in a corner or a closet, or dancing around when she has to poop)

» Hard, pellet-like poops (these are hard to pass and cause pain)

» Super-loose poop (which can ooze past longer, hard poops stuck inside the large intestines)

- » XXXL poops (means she has been holding it in for a long time)

- » "Skid marks" in her underwear (from holding in the poop)

- » Little flecks of blood in the poop (from hard poop scraping against her intestine)

- » Demanding to poop in a pull-up rather than the toilet

If you try to start potty training while your child is constipated, you'll get nothing but frustration. It's best to delay potty training until your child is no longer constipated.

Unfortunately, potty training can sometimes cause a bit of constipation because your child isn't yet comfortable enough on the toilet to poop freely, so she may hold it for extra long. Usually, kids will go two days before pooping during potty training. If it goes much longer than that, consult with your pediatrician until your child is pooping soft, mushy stools on a regular basis.

One way to help your child feel comfortable pooping on the potty is to show her that poop is always supposed to go inside the toilet, instead of being wrapped in her diaper/pull-up like a piece of trash. Change your child in the bathroom when accidents occur. If it's a poop accident, dump the poops in the toilet, let her take a peek inside, and then let her flush. I know this sounds weird, but I promise you it really helps.

After age four, if your child is showing signs of constipation, consult with your pediatrician. She may have something called functional constipation, and you'll want a doctor to take a look.

STEP 5:
keep teaching

YAY, YOU'VE GOTTEN ALMOST TO THE END of this potty-training plan, and hopefully it was successful! After three days of potty training, you should have laid a great foundation. Now all you have to do is continue to follow through and give positive reinforcement. With each passing day, this should become easier and easier, and, once your child is four years old, she should require minimal assistance in the bathroom.

We never stop teaching our children, so other things you can teach them include:

>> How to step up to the toilet themselves

>> How to wipe themselves

>> The proper way to wash their hands

>> How to pull up their underwear and pants

You're about to be amazed at the transformation your child achieves. Parents tell me how big their child looks now that she is potty trained, and your child is about to show you how big of a kid she really is now.

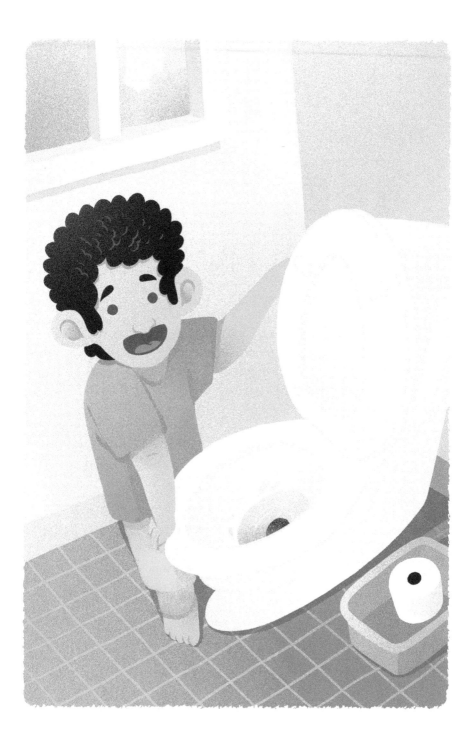

RESOURCES

Use the following resources to learn more about strategies for potty training.

AUSTIN DIAPER BANK: www.austindiapers.org

BEDWETTING AND ACCIDENTS: www.bedwettingandaccidents.com

GARY CHAPMAN'S 5 LOVE LANGUAGES: www.5lovelanguages.com

HELP A MOTHER OUT DIAPER BANK: www.helpamotherout.org

LOVE AND LOGIC: www.loveandlogic.com

YOUR VILLAGE CONSULTING: www.yourvillageconsulting.com

DR. DAUM'S WEBSITE: www.doctordaum.com

THE ENCOPRESIS CENTER: www.encopresiscenter.com

INDEX

About the Author

BRANDI BRUCKS, CPST, is the Director of Your Village Consulting in Austin, Texas. As a Potty Training Consultant and Behavior Specialist, she potty trains children as young as 21 months up to 4 years old. She also helps children correct sleep issues and establish healthy sleeping habits. She holds a Master's Degree in Elementary Education from Simmons College in Boston, Massachusetts.

About the Foreword Author

DR. FREDRIC DAUM is a Harvard graduate with 45 years of experience in Pediatric Gastroenterology. He is Chief of Pediatric Gastroenterology at Winthrop University Hospital in Mineola, New York, and Professor of Pediatrics and Clinical Scholar in the School of Medicine at Stony Brook University. He is world renowned for his treatment of stool withholding and encopresis.

CPSIA information can be obtained
at www.ICGtesting.com
Printed in the USA
JSHW011957280220
4526JS00001B/1

9 781623 157906